Intermittent Fasting 101

101

Embrace A New Lifestyle And Reach Your Weight Loss Goals With Fast-Friendly, Kitchen-Tested Recipes

Thalia Field

TABLE OF CONTENTS

INTRODUCTION

This book is divided into small chapters where you will learn what the plan brings, what you should eat when fasting and how to start intermittent fasting. This book will cookbook you through a short introduction - a cookbook to why you should start intermittent fasting, a step-by-step cookbook for beginners who intermittently fast, and tips on how to incorporate it into your routine. I have created 3 Lent schedules that you can use according to your goals. Contains a list of fasting times to use when shopping, along with a list of what to eat during the day and when and where.

Method 16-8, which is a daily intermittent fast, includes a 24-hour fast. This extended fasting period allows the body to remain in a fat and burn state for a longer period compared to the daily or weekly schedule for intermittent fasting.

If you are not planning on doing a 24-hour fast, I suggest starting with a 12-hour fast once or twice a week and doing it frequently. If you think intermittent fasting is the way to go, I would recommend eating low and slow for the first few days or weeks of Lent. However, if you are eating low in calories and want to try intermittent fasting, we recommend sticking to what you eat (i.e. eating only 8).

The most popular form of intermittent fasting is the 16: 8 method, which limits the daily meal time to 8 hours, not 24 hours. The Leangain model of intermittent fasting is usually followed, using a 16-hour fast followed by an 8-hour meal over a period of time. Finally, warrior fasting involves eating only one meal a day for 8-12 hours after a 20 / 4 / 20 hour fast. The most commonly used form of long-term fasting (i.e. fasting for 20, 4 or 20 hours) is also the "16: 8 Method," because it involves a fasting time of about 16 hours and means that the window of eating is spread over eight hours and you do not eat for all of these 24 hours.

In other words, interval fasting is a form of long-term fasting, in which one abstains from food for a certain period of time.

In order to take advantage of all the benefits of intermittent fasting, you must fast for at least 12 hours, but there is a better way to intermittent fasting, so that you can start fasting for a longer period, such as 2-3 weeks. If you stick to your self-imposed fasting schedule and fast for 2 or 3 weeks, you will adapt and have similar energy levels during the fasting window, regardless of whether you fast for 2, 3, 4, 5, 6, 7, 8 or 10 days.

Here are some more intensive methods of intermittent fasting, and I have created 3 fasting schedules that you can use depending on your goals. Adherence to these two routines is often associated with fasting and intermittent fasting, but is not really a fasting program. Intermittent fasting for beginners: There are flexible intermittent fasting schedules, which include a 14-16 hour fast, typically associated with circadian rhythms. You have the option to start quickly and limit the duration to 2-3 weeks or a longer period.

Intermittent fasting is really a lifestyle choice, where you eat for a set period of time and fast for the rest of the time. There are people who skip breakfast, which means that you can usually eat lunch and early dinner before the cycle starts again. If you plan your meals within a set period of time, intermittent fasting can go begging, and that's remarkably simple. Whether you fast daily or intermittently, you simply learn that it is the same: you do not eat during mealtime, but you do not eat after mealtime - in time; you simply eat as if you were fasting.

If you are considering trying intermittent fasting, here are a few types of intermittent fasting plans you can follow. If you are already on a keto diet, you will find that fasting outside the window with an intermittent fasting plan is easier to manage than a daily or daily diet.

Intermittent fasting is one of them, but the best part is that it's not a diet plan, it's a lifestyle plan. This Keto Beginners Plan offers you an easy - user-friendly, low-carb - and healthy way to practice intermittent fasting. Intermittent fasting plans go a step further by creating a "lifestyle" of fasting that is high in fat - and offers benefits in terms of burning. You can practice your intermittent fasting in various ways, from a regular diet to an intermittent diet or even a combination of both. You can also practice it daily or weekly for a few weeks or months.

BREAKFAST RECIPES

1. Coconutty Cereal

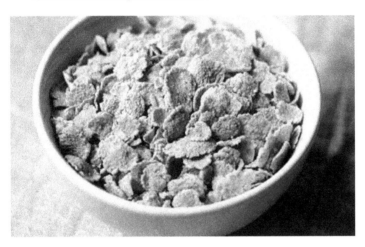

Preparation Time: 5 minutes

Cooking Time: 5 minutes

Servings: 2

Ingredients:

- cup coconut, shredded or flakes
- 1 teaspoon erythritol
- Unsweetened nondairy milk of choice (I use macadamia milk), for serving

Directions:

1. .Preheat the oven to 350°F.
2. On a baking sheet, arrange the coconut flakes in a single layer.
3. Bake for about 5 minutes, until nice and golden.

4. Allow the coconut flakes cool for around 5 to 10 minutes, then toss them with the erythritol in a plastic zip top bag and shake.
5. Divide between two bowls and pour in the nondairy milk. Serve.

Nutrition: Calories: 247 Total Fat: 24g Protein: 3g Total Carbs: 7g Fiber: 6g Net Carbs: 1g

2. Buckwheat Spaghetti with Chicken Cabbage and Savory Food Recipes in Mass Sauce

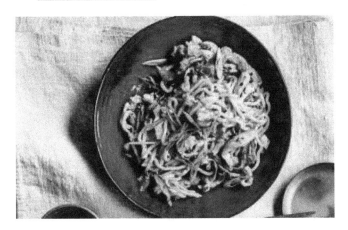

Preparation Time: 15 minutes

Cooking Time: 15 minutes'

Servings: 2

Ingredients:

- For the noodles:
- 2-3 handfuls of cabbage leaves (removed from the stem and cut)
- Buckwheat noodles 150g / 5oz (100% buckwheat, without wheat)
- 3-4 shiitake mushrooms, sliced
- 1 teaspoon of coconut oil or butter
- 1 brown onion, finely chopped
- 1 medium chicken breast, sliced or diced

- 1 long red pepper, thinly sliced (seeds in or out depending on how hot you like it)
- 2 large garlic cloves, diced
- 2-3 tablespoons of Tamari sauce (gluten-free soy sauce)
- For the miso dressing:
- 1 tablespoon and a half of fresh organic miso
- 1 tablespoon of Tamari sauce
- 1 tablespoon of extra virgin olive oil
- 1 tablespoon of lemon or lime juice
- 1 teaspoon of sesame oil (optional)

Directions:

1. Boil a medium saucepan of water. Add the black cabbage and cook 1 minute, until it is wilted. Remove and reserve, but reserve the water and return to boiling. Add your soba noodles and cook according to the directions on the package (usually about 5 minutes). Rinse with cold water and reserve.

2. In the meantime, fry the shiitake mushrooms in a little butter or coconut oil (about a teaspoon) for 2-3 minutes, until its color is lightly browned on each side. Sprinkle with sea salt and reserve.

3. In that same pan, heat more coconut oil or lard over medium-high heat. Fry the onion and chili for 2-3 minutes, and then add the chicken pieces. Cook 5 minutes on medium heat, stirring a few times, then add the garlic, tamari sauce, and a little water. Cook for

another 2-3 minutes, stirring continuously until your chicken is cooked.

4. Finally, add the cabbage and soba noodles and stir the chicken to warm it.

5. Stir the miso sauce and sprinkle the noodles at the end of the cooking, in this way you will keep alive all the beneficial probiotics in the miso.

Nutrition: 305 calories Fat 11 Fiber 7 Carbs 9 Protein 12

3. Baked Omelet with Bacon

Preparation Time: 5 minutes

Cooking Time: 30 minutes

Servings: 1

Ingredients:

- 4 eggs
- 140 g diced bacon
- 85 g butter
- 60 g fresh spinach
- tbsp. l finely chopped fresh onions (to taste)
- salt and pepper

Directions:

1. Preheat the oven to 400 ° F. Oil one small baking dish (per serving).
2. Fry the bacon and spinach in the remaining oil.
3. In another bowl, whisk the eggs until it's foamy. Mix the bacon and spinach, gradually adding the fat remaining after frying the products.
4. Then add finely chopped onions. Flavor the dish with salt and pepper.
5. Put the mixture into a baking sheet then bake for at least 20 minutes or until golden brown.
6. Recover the dish and let it cool for a few minutes. After that, you can serve.

Nutrition: Carbohydrates: 12 g Fats: 72 g Proteins: 21 g Calories: 737

4. Egg Intermittent Cupcakes

Preparation Time: 10 minutes

Cooking Time: 25 minutes

Servings: 6

Ingredients:

- 2 pcs green onions finely chopped green onions
- 150 g Sausages of sliced sausages or bacon
- 12 pcs Egg
- 2 tbsp. 1 Pesto
- Salt and pepper
- 175 g grated cheese

Directions:

1. Preheat the oven to 350 ° F.
2. Lubricate the muffin pan with butter.
3. Fill onions and sausages at the bottom of the molds.
4. Beat the eggs with pesto, salt, and pepper. Add cheese and mix thoroughly.
5. Fill the cupcake pan with the resulting mixture.
6. Bake in the oven for 15-20 minutes depending on the size of the mold.

Nutrition: Carbohydrates: 2 g Fats: 26 g Proteins: 23 g Kcal: 336

5. Sandwiches with Salad

Preparation Time: 5 minutes

Cooking Time: 0 minutes

Servings: 1

Ingredients:

- 50 g Roman salad
- 15 g Butter
- 30 g Cheese of Eden cheese or other cheese (to your taste)
- 0.5 pcs Avocado
- pc cherry tomato

Directions:

1. Rinse the lettuce leaves thoroughly and use them as a base for the filling.
2. Oil the leaves, chop the cheese, avocado, and tomato and place on the leaves.

Nutrition: Fats: 34 g Proteins: 10 g Carbohydrates: 3 g Calories: 374

6. Intermittent Avocado with Bacon

Preparation Time: 5 minutes

Cooking Time: 20 minutes

Servings: 1

Ingredients:

- 4 hard-boiled egg
- pc avocado
- tbsp. olive oil
- 100 g bacon
- salt and pepper

Directions:

1. Preheat oven to 350 ° F.
2. In a pan that filled of water, put the egg. Set to a boil and let it brew for 8-10 minutes. Place the eggs in ice water immediately after preparation to make them easier to clean.
3. Cut the eggs in half and dig up the yolks. Place them in a small bowl.
4. Add avocado, butter, and mashed potatoes until salt and pepper are mixed to taste.
5. Set the bacon on a baking sheet then bake until crispy. It takes about 5-7 minutes.
6. Using a spoon, carefully add the mixture back to the cooked egg whites and set the sails with bacon! Enjoy it!

Nutrition: Pure carbohydrates: 1 g Fats: 13 g Proteins: 5 g Calories: 144

7. Intermittent Omelet with Mushrooms

Preparation Time: 5 minutes

Cooking Time: 10 minutes

Servings: 1

Ingredients:

- 3 eggs
- 30 g butter for frying
- 30 g (60 ml) grated cheese
- 1/5 onion
- 3 pcs. mushrooms
- salt and pepper

Directions:

1. Break the eggs then put the contents into a small bowl.
2. Add salt and pepper to taste.
3. Beat the eggs with a fork until a uniform foam is formed.
4. In a pan, heat a piece of butter, and as soon as the butter has melted, pour the egg mixture into the pan.
5. When the mixture begins to harden and fry, and the eggs on top will still be liquid, sprinkle them with cheese, mushrooms, and onions (to taste).
6. Take a spatula and gently pry the edges of the omelet on one side, and then fold the omelet in half. As soon as the dish begins to take a golden brownish tint, remove the pan from the stove then place the omelet on a plate.

Nutrition: Carbohydrates: 5 g Fats: 44 g Proteins: 26 g Kcal: 649

8. Cacao Crunch Cereal

Preparation Time: 5 minutes

Cooking Time: 0 minutes

Servings: 2

Ingredients:

- ½ cup slivered almonds
- 2 tablespoons coconut, shredded or flakes
- 2 tablespoons chia seeds
- 2 tablespoons cacao nibs
- 2 tablespoons sunflower seeds
- Unsweetened nondairy milk of choice (I use macadamia milk), for serving

Directions:

1. In a small bowl, mix the almonds, coconut, chia seeds, cacao nibs, and sunflower seeds. Divide between two bowls.
2. Pour in the nondairy milk and serve.

Nutrition: Calories: 325 Total Fat: 27 Protein: 10g Total Carbs: 17g Fiber: 12g Net Carbs: 5g

LUNCH RECIPES

9. Shrimp with Linguine

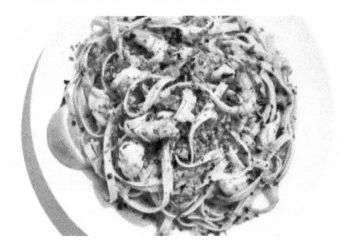

Preparation Time: 10 minutes

Cooking Time: 10 minutes

Servings: 4

Ingredients:

- lb. Shrimp, cleaned
- 1 lb. Linguine
- 1 tbsp Butter
- ½ cup white Wine
- ½ cup Parmesan cheese, shredded
- Garlic cloves, minced
- 1 cup Parsley, chopped
- Salt and Pepper, to taste
- ½ cup Coconut Cream, for garnish
- ½ Avocado, diced, for garnish

- tbsp fresh Dill, for garnish

Directions:

1. Melt the butter on Sauté. Stir in linguine, garlic cloves and parsley. Cook for 4 minutes until aromatic. Add shrimp and white wine; season with salt and pepper, seal the lid.
2. Select Manual and cook for 5 minutes on High pressure. When ready, quick release the pressure. Unseal and remove the lid. Press Sauté, add the cheese and stir well until combined, for 30-40 seconds. Serve topped with the coconut cream, avocado, and dill.

Nutrition: Calories 412, Protein 48g, Net Carbs 5.6g, Fat 21g

10. Mexican Cod Fillets

Preparation Time: 10 minutes

Cooking Time: 10 minutes

Servings: 3

Ingredients:

- 3 Cod fillets
- Onion, sliced
- cups Cabbage
- Juice from 1 Lemon
- 1 Jalapeno Pepper
- ½ tsp Oregano
- ½ tsp Cumin powder
- ½ tsp Cayenne Pepper
- tbsp Olive oil
- Salt and black Pepper to taste

Directions:

1. Heat the oil on Sauté, and add onion, cabbage, lemon juice, jalapeño pepper, cayenne pepper, cumin powder and oregano, and stir to combine. Cook for 8-10 minutes.

2. Season with salt and black pepper. Arrange the cod fillets in the sauce, using a spoon to cover each piece with some of the sauce. Seal the lid and press Manual. Cook for 5 minutes on High pressure. When ready, do a quick release and serve.

Nutrition: Calories 306, Protein 21g, Net Carbs 6.8g, Fat 19.4g

11. Simple Mushroom Chicken Mix

Preparation Time: 5 minutes

Cooking Time: 18 minutes

Servings: 2

Ingredients:

- 2 Tomatoes, chopped
- ½ lb. Chicken, cooked and mashed
- cup Broccoli, chopped
- 1 tbsp Butter
- tbsp Mayonnaise
- ½ cup Mushroom soup
- Salt and Pepper, to taste
- 1 Onion, sliced

Directions:

1. Once cooked, put the chicken into a bowl. In a separate bowl, mix the mayo, mushroom soup, tomatoes, onion, broccoli, and salt and pepper. Add the chicken.
2. Grease a round baking tray with butter. Put the mixture in a tray. Add 2 cups of water into the Instant Pot and place the trivet inside. Place the tray on top. Seal the lid, press Manual and cook for 14 minutes on High pressure. When ready, do a quick release.

Nutrition: Calories 561, Protein 28.5g, Net Carbs 6.3g, Fat 49.5g

12. Squash Spaghetti with Bolognese Sauce

Preparation Time: 5 minutes

Cooking Time: 10 minutes

Servings: 3

Ingredients:

- large Squash, cut into 2 and seed pulp removed
- cups Water
- Bolognese Sauce to serve

Directions:

1. Place the trivet and add the water. Add in the squash, seal the lid, select Manual and cook on High Pressure for 8 minutes. Once ready, quickly release the pressure. Carefully remove the squash; use two forks to shred the inner skin. Serve with Bolognese sauce.

Nutrition: Calories 37, Protein 0.9g, Net Carbs 7.8g, Fat 0.4g

13. Healthy Halibut Fillets

Preparation Time: 5 minutes

Cooking Time: 10 minutes

Servings: 2

Ingredients:

- 2 Halibut fillets
- tbsp Dill
- 1 tbsp Onion powder
- 1 cup Parsley, chopped
- tbsp Paprika
- 1 tbsp Garlic powder
- 1 tbsp Lemon Pepper
- tbsp Lemon juice

Directions:

1. Mix lemon juice, lemon pepper, garlic powder, and paprika, parsley, dill and onion powder in a bowl. Pour the mixture in the Instant pot and place the halibut fish over it.
2. Seal the lid, press Manual mode and cook for 10 minutes on High pressure. When ready, do a quick pressure release by setting the valve to venting.

Nutrition: Calories 283, Protein 22.5g, Net Carbs 6.2g, Fat 16.4g

14. Clean Salmon with Soy Sauce

Preparation Time: 10 minutes

Cooking Time: 30 minutes

Servings: 2

Ingredients:

- 2 Salmon fillets
- 2 tbsp Avocado oil
- 2 tbsp Soy sauce
- tbsp Garlic powder
- 1 tbsp fresh Dill to garnish
- Salt and Pepper, to taste

Directions:

1. To make the marinade, thoroughly mix the soy sauce, avocado oil, salt, pepper and garlic powder into a bowl. Dip salmon in the mixture and place in the refrigerator for 20 minutes.
2. Transfer the contents to the Instant pot. Seal, set on Manual and cook for 10 minutes on high pressure. When ready, do a quick release. Serve topped with the fresh dill.

Nutrition: Calories 512, Protein 65g, Net Carbs 3.2g, Fat 21g

15. Simple Salmon with Eggs

Preparation Time: 2 minutes

Cooking Time: 5 minutes

Servings: 3

Ingredients:

- lb. Salmon, cooked, mashed
- Eggs, whisked
- Onions, chopped
- 2 stalks celery, chopped
- 1 cup Parsley, chopped
- 1 tbsp Olive oil
- Salt and Pepper, to taste

Directions:

1. Mix salmon, onion, celery, parsley, and salt and pepper, in a bowl. Form into 6 patties about 1 inch thick and dip them in the whisked eggs. Heat oil in the Instant pot on Sauté mode.
2. Add the patties to the pot and cook on both sides, for about 5 minutes and transfer to the plate. Allow to cool and serve.

Nutrition: Calories 331, Protein 38g, Net Carbs 5.3g, Fat 16g

16. Easy Shrimp

Preparation Time: 4 minutes

Cooking Time: 5 minutes

Servings: 2

Ingredients:

- lb. Shrimp, peeled and deveined
- Garlic cloves, crushed
- 1 tbsp Butter.
- A pinch of red Pepper
- Salt and Pepper, to taste
- 1 cup Parsley, chopped

Directions:

1. Melt butter on Sauté mode. Add shrimp, garlic, red pepper, salt and pepper. Cook for 5 minutes, stirring occasionally the shrimp until pink. Serve topped with parsley.

Nutrition: Calories 245, Protein 45g, Net Carbs 4.8g, Fat 4g

17. Scallops with Mushroom Special

Preparation Time: 15 minutes

Cooking Time: 20 minutes

Servings: 2

Ingredients:

- lb. Scallops
- Onions, chopped
- 1 tbsp Butter
- tbsp Olive oil
- 1 cup Mushrooms
- Salt and Pepper, to taste
- 1 tbsp Lemon juice
- ½ cup Whipping Cream
- 1 tbsp chopped fresh Parsley

Directions:

1. Heat the oil on Sauté. Add onions, butter, mushrooms, salt and pepper. Cook for 3 to 5 minutes. Add the lemon juice and scallops. Lock the lid and set to Manual mode.
2. Cook for 15 minutes on High pressure. When ready, do a quick pressure release and carefully open the lid. Top with a drizzle of cream and fresh parsley.

Nutrition: Calories 312, Protein 31g, Net Carbs 7.3g, Fat 10.4g

18. Delicious Creamy Crab Meat

Preparation Time: 5 minutes

Cooking Time: 10 minutes

Servings: 3

Ingredients:

- lb. Crab meat
- ½ cup Cream cheese
- tbsp Mayonnaise
- Salt and Pepper, to taste
- 1 tbsp Lemon juice
- 1 cup Cheddar cheese, shredded

Directions:

1. Mix mayo, cream cheese, salt and pepper, and lemon juice in a bowl. Add in crab meat and make small balls. Place the balls inside the pot. Seal the lid and press Manual.
2. Cook for 10 minutes on High pressure. When done, allow the pressure to release naturally for 10 minutes. Sprinkle the cheese over and serve!

Nutrition: Calories 443, Protein 41g, Net Carbs 2.5g, Fat 30.4g

SIDE DISHES

19. Instant Zucchini with Green Peppercorn Sauce

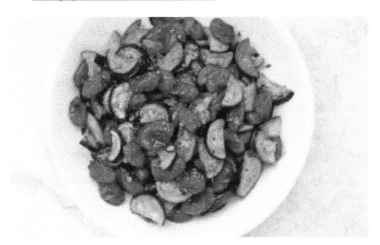

Preparation Time: 2 minutes

Cooking Time: 10 minutes

Servings: 4

Ingredients:

- cup water
- zucchini, sliced
- Sea salt, to taste
- Green Peppercorn Sauce:
- tablespoons butter
- 1/2 cup green onions, minced
- 2 tablespoons Cognac
- ½ cups chicken broth
- cup whipping cream

- ½ tablespoons green peppercorns in brine, drained and crushed slightly

Directions:

1. Add water and a steamer basket to the Instant Pot. Arrange your zucchini on the steamer basket.
2. Secure the lid. Choose "Manual" mode and Low pressure; cook for 3 minutes. Once cooking is complete, use a quick pressure release; carefully remove the lid.
3. Season zucchini with salt and set aside.
4. Wipe down the Instant Pot with a damp cloth. Press the "Sauté" button to heat up your Instant Pot.
5. Melt the butter and then, sauté green onions until tender. Add Cognac and cook for 2 minutes longer. Then, pour in chicken broth and let it boil another 4 minutes.
6. Lastly, stir in the cream and peppercorns. Continue to simmer until the sauce is thickened and thoroughly warmed.
7. Serve your zucchini with the sauce on the side. Bon appétit!

Nutrition: 251 Calories; 15.3g Fat; 3.2g Total Carbs; 20.2g Protein; 1.5g Sugars

20. Lazy Sunday Mushroom Ragoût

Preparation Time: 2 minutes

Cooking Time: 10 minutes

Servings: 4

Ingredients:

- 3 tablespoons butter, at room temperature
- 1/2 cup white onions, peeled and sliced
- cup chicken sausage, casing removed, sliced
- pound Chanterelle mushrooms, sliced
- stalks spring garlic, diced
- Kosher salt and ground black pepper, to taste
- 1/2 teaspoon red pepper flakes
- tablespoons tomato paste
- 1/2 cup good Pinot Noir
- cup chicken stock
- 1/2 cup double cream
- tablespoons fresh chives, chopped

Directions:

1. Press the "Sauté" button to heat up your Instant Pot. Once hot, melt the butter and sauté the onions until tender and translucent.
2. Add the sausage and mushrooms; continue to sauté until the sausage is no longer pink and the mushrooms are fragrant.
3. Then, stir in garlic and cook it for 30 to 40 seconds more or until aromatic. Now, add the salt, black pepper, red pepper, tomato paste, Pinot Noir, and chicken stock.

4. Secure the lid. Choose "Manual" mode and High pressure; cook for 5 minutes. Once cooking is complete, use a quick pressure release; carefully remove the lid.
5. After that, add double cream and press the "Sauté" button. Continue to simmer until everything is heated through and slightly thickened.
6. Lastly, divide your stew among individual bowls; top with fresh chopped chives and serve warm.

Nutrition: 279 Calories; 22.3g Fat; 6.3g Total Carbs; 8.7g Protein; 3.2g Sugars

MEATS RECIPES

21. Smoked Lamb

Preparation Time: 30 minutes + smoke time

Cooking Time: 100 minutes

Servings: 4

Ingredients:

- 2.5kg boneless 5 lb. shoulder
- 3-4 sprigs fresh rosemary
- Himalayan salt
- Freshly ground black pepper
- About 6 cups of cherry wood chips

Directions:

1. Place 4 cups of wood chips to soak in water for at least an hour before smoking your lamb.
2. Remove the fillet around the shoulder of lamb, rinse it in cold water and dry it. Place the lamb on a cutting board (cut the thicker parts if necessary) and make several deep incisions along with the meat with a kitchen knife. Insert pieces of fresh rosemary into these incisions. Sprinkle generously with salt and pepper.
3. Preheat your outdoor grill to 225 ° F. Lighting a single burner in the lowest setting should be the trick.
4. Make 8 bags of wood chips. Cut a piece of heavy-duty 12 "x 24" aluminum foil for each bag (double if you are using lighter weight paper) and place about half a cup

of damp wood chips at 1 end of the paper. Add a handful of dried chips and fold the sheet over the wood chips. Fold the 4 edges in the center at least twice, then make holes in the top and bottom of the bag with a fork or other sharp object.

5. Lift the grill on the ignition element and place 2 bags directly on the heat source. Close and wait for the smoke to come out of the bags.

6. Place the roast lamb on the other side of the grill and close the lid.

7. Smoke the meat for about 6 hours and replace the bags with 2 new 1s every 90 min If necessary, increase the heat under the new bag until the smoke comes out and lower the temperature.

8. Try to keep the temperature of your grill as stable as possible at around 225 ° F. *Please note that it is not necessary to get massive amounts of smoke to get a good taste however if you feel you don't have enough, no contact to add more dry chips to your foil pouches or place an aluminum container with a handful of baked chips next to your existing foil pouches.*

9. When the lamb has smoked for 6 hours, remove it from the grill and wrap it in aluminum foil. Use a double layer to make sure n1 of the cooking juices leak out. You want to preserve moisture at this time.

10. Place it back on the grill and crank up the heat to 350° F. Cook the meat for another 90 min, or until the meat becomes very tender and can be easily removed with a fork.

11. Take off the roast from the grill, then let it sit for 10 min, then cut and serve sprinkled with the cooking juices.

Nutrition: Calories: 797 kcal Protein: 136.98 g Fat: 27.1 g Carbohydrates: 1.97 g

22. Lamb Souvlaki

Preparation Time: 15 minutes + marinate time

Cooking Time: 45 minutes

Servings: 2

Ingredients:

- 2 lbs. of Fat-free lamb, cut into 1-inch pieces
- 2 lemon juice
- 3 tbsp. olive oil
- ½ tsp salt
- ½ tsp freshly ground pepper
- tbsp. dried oregano
- garlic cloves, finely chopped
- medium onion, thinly sliced

Directions:

1. Combine olive oil, lemon juice, salt, pepper, oregano, garlic, and onion in a large bowl. Place the slices of meat in the pan and mix so that the meat is completely covered with marinade. Cover and let cool for a minimum of 2 hours and a maximum of 24 hours. Bring chicken on metal or bamboo skewers.
2. Roast the skewer on all sides until golden.
3. Serve with pita bread.

Nutrition: Calories: 1396 kcal Protein: 114.74 g Fat: 99.7 g Carbohydrates: 4.23 g

23. Lamb Saagwali

Preparation Time: 15 minutes

Cooking Time: 50 minutes

Servings: 4

Ingredients:

- 2 to 3 lb. of Fat-free lamb, cut into 1-inch cubes
- 4 tbsp. ghee, divided
- 2 dried red peppers
- 3 teeth
- 1-inch cinnamon stick
- 4 green cardamom pods
- tbsp. coriander seeds
- tsp cumin seeds
- large onion, diced
- tsp ginger and garlic paste
- ½ tsp turmeric
- tomatoes, diced
- 6 cups of spinach or a mixture of vegetables (mustard, kale, etc.)
- tsp coriander powder
- tsp cumin powder
- tbsp. ground kasoori methi
- ½ tsp garam masala powder
- ¼ cup cream
- salt and pepper to taste

Directions:

1. Heat 2 tbsp. ghee in a heavy-bottomed pan. Brown the lamb cubes and place them in a pressure cooker *. Cook up to 6-8 whistles. Remove from heat and set aside for steam to escape.
2. In the same pan used to brown the meat, add the red peppers, cinnamon, cardamom, and cloves. Jump until you smell it.
3. Add the coriander seeds and cumin seeds. As soon as they start to crack, add the onions.
4. Fry the onions until its almost golden.
5. Add ginger and garlic paste and turmeric. Cook until the rough odor disappears.
6. Cover and simmer until the tomatoes are tender. Add the vegetables. Thoroughly mix the vegetables and simmer for 5 min
7. Transfer to a blender. Mix until smooth.
8. Heat the remaining ghee in the previous pan and add the mixed vegetable mixture. Add the coriander, cumin and methi kasuri.
9. Cover and simmer for ten min Adjust the salt if necessary.
10. Cover and simmer the lamb for another 20 min, stirring frequently. Add water if necessary.
11. Add the cream and garam masala. Serve hot

Nutrition: Calories: 926 kcal Protein: 72.1 g Fat: 58.74 g Carbohydrates: 33 g

POULTRY

24. Traditional Hungarian Gulyás

Preparation Time: 10 minutes

Cooking Time: 1 hour and 10 minutes

Servings: 4

Ingredients:

- 1/2 cup celery ribs, chopped
- ripe tomato, pureed
- tablespoon spice mix for goulash
- (1-ounce) slices bacon, chopped
- 1/2 pound duck legs, skinless and boneless

Directions:

1. Heat a heavy-bottomed pot over the medium-high flame; then, fry the bacon for about 3 minutes. Stir in the duck legs and continue to cook until they are nicely browned on all sides.
2. Shred the meat and discard the bones. Set aside.
3. In the pan drippings, sauté the celery for about 3 minutes, stirring with a wide spatula. Add in pureed tomatoes and spice mix for goulash; add in the reserved bacon and meat.
4. Pour 2 cups of water or chicken broth into the pot.
5. Place heat to medium-low, cover, and simmer for 50 minutes more or until everything is cooked thoroughly. Serve warm and enjoy!

Nutrition: 363 Calories 22.3g Fat 5.1g Carbs 33.2g Protein 1.4g Fiber

25. Greek Chicken Stifado

Preparation Time: 10 minutes

Cooking Time: 35 minutes

Servings: 2

Ingredients:

- 2 ounces bacon, diced
- teaspoon poultry seasoning mix
- vine-ripe tomatoes, pureed
- 3/4 pound whole chicken, boneless and chopped
- 1/2 medium-sized leek, chopped

Directions:

1. Cook the bacon in the preheated skillet over medium-high heat. Fold in the chicken and continue to cook for 5 minutes more until it is no longer pink; set aside.
2. In the same skillet, sauté the leek until it has softened or about 4 minutes. Stir in the poultry seasoning mix and 2 cups of water or chicken broth.
3. Now, reduce the heat to medium-low and continue to simmer for 15 to 20 minutes.
4. Add in tomatoes along with the reserved meat. Continue to cook for a further 13 minutes or until cooked through. Bon appétit!

Nutrition: 352 Calories 14.3g Fat 5.9g Carbs 44.2g Protein 2.4g Fiber

26. Tangy Chicken with Scallions

Preparation Time: 10 minutes

Cooking Time: 40 minutes

Servings: 4

Ingredients:

- 3 tablespoons butter, melted
- pound chicken drumettes
- tablespoons white wine
- garlic clove, sliced
- tablespoon fresh scallions, chopped

Directions:

1. Arrange the chicken drumettes on a foil-lined baking pan. Brush with melted butter.
2. Add in the garlic and wine. Spice with salt and black pepper to taste. Bake in the preheated oven at 400 degrees F for about 30 minutes or until internal temperature reaches about 165 degrees F.
3. Serve garnished with scallions and enjoy!

Nutrition: 209 Calories 12.2g Fat 0.4g Carbs 23.2g Protein 1.9g Fiber

27. Double Cheese Italian Chicken

Preparation Time: 10 minutes

Cooking Time: 20 minutes

Servings: 2

Ingredients:

- 2 chicken drumsticks
- 2 cups baby spinach
- teaspoon Italian spice mix
- 1/2 cup cream cheese
- cup Asiago cheese, grated

Directions:

1. In a saucepan, heat 1 tbsp. of oil over medium-high heat. Sear the chicken drumsticks for 7 to 8 minutes or until nicely browned on all sides; reserve.
2. Pour in 1/2 cup of chicken bone broth; add in spinach and continue to cook for 5 minutes more until spinach has wilted.
3. Add in Italian spice mix, cream cheese, Asiago cheese, and reserved chicken drumsticks; partially cover and continue to cook for 5 more minutes. Serve warm.

Nutrition: 589 Calories 46g Fat 5.8g Carbs 37.5g Protein 2g Fiber

SEAFOOD RECIPES

28. Herbed Coconut Milk Steamed Mussels

Preparation Time: 10 minutes

Cooking Time: 15 minutes

Servings: 4

Ingredients:

- 2 tablespoons coconut oil
- ½ sweet onion, chopped
- 2 teaspoons minced garlic
- teaspoon grated fresh ginger
- ½ teaspoon turmeric
- cup coconut milk
- Juice of 1 lime
- 1½ pounds fresh mussels, scrubbed and debearded
- scallion, finely chopped
- tablespoons chopped fresh cilantro
- tablespoon chopped fresh thyme

Directions:

1. Sauté the aromatics. In a huge skillet, warm the coconut oil. Add the onion, garlic, ginger, and turmeric and sauté until they have softened, about 3 minutes.
2. Add the liquid. Mix in the coconut milk, lime juice then bring the mixture to a boil.

3. Steam the mussels. Put the mussels to the skillet, cover, and steam until the shells are open, about 10 minutes. Take the skillet off the heat and throw out any unopened mussels.Add the herbs. Stir in the scallion, cilantro, and thyme.Serve. Divide the mussels and the sauce into 4 bowls and serve them immediately.

Nutrition: Calories: 319 Total fat: 23g Total carbs: 8g Fiber: 2g; Net carbs: 6g Sodium: 395mg Protein: 23g

29. Basil Halibut Red Pepper Packets

Preparation Time: 10 minutes

Cooking Time: 20 minutes

Servings: 4

Ingredients:

- 2 cups cauliflower florets
- cup roasted red pepper strips
- ½ cup sliced sun-dried tomatoes
- 4 (4-ounce) halibut fillets
- ¼ cup chopped fresh basil
- Juice of 1 lemon
- ¼ cup good-quality olive oil
- Sea salt, for seasoning
- Freshly ground black pepper, for seasoning

Directions:

1. Preheat the oven. Set the oven temperature to 400°F. Cut into four (12-inch) square pieces of aluminum foil. Have a baking sheet ready.Make the packets. Divide the cauliflower, red pepper strips, and sun-dried tomato between the four pieces of foil, placing the vegetables in the middle of each piece. Top each pile with 1 halibut fillet, and top each fillet with equal amounts of the basil, lemon juice, and olive oil. Fold and crimp the foil to form sealed packets of fish and vegetables and place them on the baking sheet.Bake. Bake the packets for about 20 minutes, until the fish flakes with a fork. Be careful of the steam when you

open the packet!Serve. Transfer the vegetables and halibut to four plates, season with salt and pepper, and serve immediately.

Nutrition: Calories: 294 Total fat: 18g Total carbs: 8g Fiber: 3g Net carbs: 5g Sodium: 114mg Protein: 25g

30. Sherry and Butter Prawns

Preparation Time: 5 minutes

Cooking Time: 5 minutes

Servings: 4

Ingredients:

- ½ pounds king prawns, peeled and deveined
- tablespoons dry sherry
- teaspoon dried basil
- 1/2 teaspoon mustard seeds
- ½ tablespoons fresh lemon juice
- teaspoon cayenne pepper, crushed
- tablespoon garlic paste
- 1/2 stick butter, at room temperature

Directions:

1. Whisk the dry sherry with cayenne pepper, garlic paste, basil, mustard seeds, lemon juice and prawns. Let it marinate for 1 hour in your refrigerator.
2. In a frying pan, melt the butter over medium-high flame, basting with the reserved marinade.
3. Sprinkle with salt and pepper to taste.

Nutrition: 294 Calories 14.3g Fat 3.6g Carbs 34.6g Protein 1.4g Fiber

31. Clams with Garlic-Tomato Sauce

Preparation Time: 5 minutes

Cooking Time: 20 minutes

Servings: 4

Ingredients:

- 40 littleneck clams
- For the Sauce:
- 2 tomatoes, pureed
- 2 tablespoons olive oil
- shallot, chopped
- Sea salt, to taste
- Freshly ground black pepper, to taste
- 1/2 teaspoon paprika
- 1/3 cup port wine
- garlic cloves, pressed
- 1/2 lemon, cut into wedges

Directions:

1. Grill the clams until they are open, for 5 to 6 minutes.
2. In a frying pan, heat the olive oil over moderate heat. Cook the shallot and garlic until tender and fragrant.
3. Stir in the pureed tomatoes, salt, black pepper and paprika and continue to cook an additional 10 to 12 minutes, up to well cooked.
4. Heat off and add in the port wine; stir to combine. Garnish with fresh lemon wedges.

Nutrition: 134 Calories 7.8g Fat 5.9g Carbs 8.3g Protein 1g Fiber

32. Amberjack Fillets with Cheese Sauce

Preparation Time: 10 minutes

Cooking Time: 10 minutes

Servings: 4

Ingredients:

- 6 amberjack fillets
- 1/4 cup fresh tarragon chopped
- 2 tablespoons olive oil, at room temperature
- Sea salt, to taste
- Ground black pepper, to taste
- For the Sauce:
- 1/3 cup vegetable broth
- 3/4 cup double cream
- 1/3 cup Romano cheese, grated
- 3 teaspoons butter, at room temperature
- 2 garlic cloves, finely minced

Directions:

1. In a non-stick frying pan, warm the olive oil until sizzling.
2. Once hot, fry the amberjack for about 6 minutes per side or until the edges are turning opaque. Sprinkle them with salt, black pepper, and tarragon. Reserve.
3. To make the sauce, melt the butter in a saucepan over moderately high heat. Sauté the garlic until tender and fragrant or about 2 minutes.
4. Add in the vegetable broth and cream and continue to cook for 5 to 6 minutes more; heat off.

5. Stir in the Romano cheese and continue stirring in the residual heat for a couple of minutes more.

Nutrition: 285 Calories 20.4g Fat 1.2g Carbs 23.8g Protein 0.1g Fiber

33. Tilapia with Spicy Dijon Sauce

Preparation Time: 10 minutes

Cooking Time: 5 minutes

Servings: 4

Ingredients:

- tablespoon butter, room temperature
- chili peppers, deveined and minced
- cup heavy cream
- teaspoon Dijon mustard
- pound tilapia fish, cubed
- Sea salt, to taste
- Ground black pepper, to taste
- cup white onions, chopped
- teaspoon garlic, pressed
- 1/2 cup dark rum

Directions:

1. Toss the tilapia with salt, pepper, onions, garlic, chili peppers and rum. Let it marinate for 2 hours in your refrigerator.
2. In a grill pan, melt the butter over a moderately high heat. Sear the fish in hot butter, basting with the reserved marinade.
3. Add in the mustard and cream and continue to cook until everything is thoroughly cooked, for 2 to 3 minutes.

Nutrition: 228 Calories 13g Fat 6.5g Carbs 13.7g Protein 1.1g Fiber

34. Garlic Butter Shrimps

Preparation Time: 13 minutes

Cooking Time: 16 minutes

Servings: 3

Ingredients:

- ½ pound shrimp, peeled and deveined
- 2 garlic cloves
- ½ white onion
- 3 tbsp. ghee butter
- tsp black pepper
- lemon (peeled)
- Himalayan rock salt to taste

Directions:

1. Preheat the oven to 425F
2. Mince the garlic and onion, cut the lemon in half
3. Season the shrimps with pink salt and pepper
4. Slice one-half of the lemon thinly, cut the other half into 2 pieces
5. Grease a baking dish with the butter; combine the shrimp with the garlic, onion and lemon slices, put in the baking dish
6. Bake the shrimps for 15 minutes, stirring halfway through
7. Remove the shrimps from the oven and squeeze the juice from 2 lemon pieces over the dish

Nutrition: Carbs: 39 g Fat: 198 g Protein: 32 g Calories: 338

35. Oven-Baked Sole Fillets

Preparation Time: 10 minutes

Cooking Time: 20 minutes

Servings: 4

Ingredients:

- 2 tablespoons olive oil
- 1/2 tablespoon Dijon mustard
- teaspoon garlic paste
- 1/2 tablespoon fresh ginger, minced
- 1/2 teaspoon porcini powder
- Salt and ground black pepper, to taste
- 1/2 teaspoon paprika
- 4 sole fillets
- 1/4 cup fresh parsley, chopped

Directions:

1. Combine the oil, Dijon mustard, garlic paste, ginger, porcini powder, salt, black pepper, and paprika.
2. Rub this mixture all over sole fillets. Place the sole fillets in a lightly oiled baking pan.
3. Bake in the preheated oven at 400 degrees F for about 20 minutes.

Nutrition: 195 Calories 8.2g Fat 0.5g Carbs 28.7g Protein 0.6g Fiber

VEGETABLES

36. Vegetable Tempeh Kabobs

Preparation Time: 10 minutes

Cooking Time: 16 minutes

Servings: 2

Ingredients:

- 10 oz tempeh, cut into chunks
- ½ cups water
- red onion, cut into chunks
- red bell pepper, cut chunks
- yellow bell pepper, cut into chunks
- tbsp. olive oil
- cup sugar-free barbecue sauce

Directions:

1. Place the water to boil in a pot over medium heat, and once it has boiled, turn the heat off, and add the tempeh. Cover the pot and let the tempeh steam for 5 minutes to remove its bitterness.
2. Drain the tempeh after. Pour the barbecue sauce in a bowl, add the tempeh to it, and coat with the sauce. Cover the bowl then marinate in the fridge for 2 hours.
3. Preheat grill to 350ºF, and thread the tempeh, yellow bell pepper, red bell pepper, and onion.
4. Brush the grate of the grill with olive oil, place the skewers on it, and brush with barbecue sauce. Cook the

kabobs for 3 minutes on each side while rotating and brushing with more barbecue sauce.

5. Once ready, transfer the kabobs to a plate and serve with lemon cauli couscous and a tomato sauce.

Nutrition: Calories 228 Fat 15g Net Carbs 3.6g Protein 13.2g

37. Asparagus and Tarragon Flan

Preparation Time: 10 minutes

Cooking Time: 55 minutes

Servings: 4

Ingredients:

- 16 asparagus, stems trimmed
- cup water
- ½ cup whipping cream
- cup almond milk
- eggs + 2 egg yolks, beaten in a bowl
- tbsp. chopped tarragon, fresh
- Salt and black pepper to taste
- A small pinch of nutmeg
- tbsp. grated Parmesan cheese
- cups water
- 2 tbsp. butter, melted
- tbsp. butter, softened

Directions:

1. Pour the water and some salt in a pot, add the asparagus, and bring them to boil over medium heat on a stovetop for 6 minutes. Drain the asparagus; cut their tips, and reserve for garnishing. Chop the remaining asparagus into small pieces.

2. In a blender, add the chopped asparagus, whipping cream, almond milk, tarragon, ½ teaspoon of salt, nutmeg, pepper, and Parmesan cheese. Process the ingredients on high speed until smooth. Pour the

mixture through a sieve into a bowl and whisk the eggs into it.

3. Preheat the oven to 350ºF. Grease the ramekins with softened butter and share the asparagus mixture among the ramekins. Pour the melted butter over each mixture and top with 2-3 asparagus tips. Pour the remaining water into a baking dish, place it in the ramekins, and insert it in the oven.

4. Bake for 45 minutes until their middle parts are no longer watery. Remove the ramekins and let cool. Garnish the flan with the asparagus tips and serve with chilled white wine.

Nutrition: Calories 264 Fat 11.6g Net Carbs 2.5g Protein 12.5g

38. Parmesan Roasted Cabbage

Preparation Time: 5 minutes

Cooking Time: 20 minutes

Servings: 4

Ingredients:

- large head green cabbage
- 4 tbsp. melted butter
- tsp garlic powder
- Salt and black pepper to taste
- cup grated Parmesan cheese
- Grated Parmesan cheese for topping
- tbsp. chopped parsley to garnish

Directions:

1. Set the oven to 400ºF, line baking sheet using foil, and grease with cooking spray.
2. Stand the cabbage and run a knife from the top to bottom to cut the cabbage into wedges. Remove stems and wilted leaves. Mix the butter, garlic, salt, and black pepper until evenly combined.
3. Brush the mixture every side of the cabbage wedges and sprinkle with Parmesan cheese.
4. Put on the baking sheet, then bake for at least 20 minutes to soften the cabbage and melt the cheese. Remove the cabbages when golden brown, plate, and sprinkle with extra cheese and parsley. Serve warm with pan-glazed tofu.

Nutrition: Calories 268 Fat 19.3g Net Carbs 4g Protein 17.5g

39. <u>Briam with Tomato Sauce</u>

Preparation Time: 10 minutes

Cooking Time: 70 minutes

Servings: 4

Ingredients:

- 3 tbsp. olive oil
- large eggplant, halved and sliced
- large onion, thinly sliced
- cloves garlic, sliced
- 5 tomatoes, diced
- rutabagas, diced
- cup sugar-free tomato sauce
- zucchinis, sliced
- ¼ cup water
- Salt and black pepper to taste
- tbsp. dried oregano
- tbsp. chopped parsley

Directions:

1. Preheat the oven to 400ºF. Warm the olive oil in a skillet at medium heat and cook the eggplant in for 6 minutes until on the edges. After, remove to a medium bowl. Sauté the onion and garlic in the oil for 3 minutes and add them to the eggplants. Turn the heat off.

2. In the eggplant bowl, mix in the tomatoes, rutabagas, tomato sauce, and zucchinis. Add the water and stir in the salt, black pepper, oregano, and parsley. Pour the mixture in the casserole dish. Place the dish in the oven

and bake for 45 to 60 minutes. Serve the briam warm on a bed of cauli rice.

Nutrition: Calories: 365 Fat 12g, Net Carbs 12.5g Protein 11.3g

SOUPS AND STEWS

40. Egg Broth

Preparation Time: 5 minutes

Cooking Time: 5 minutes

Servings: 4

Ingredients:

- 2 tablespoons unsalted butter
- 4 cups chicken broth
- 3 large eggs
- Salt and black pepper, to taste
- 1 sliced green onion, for garnish

Directions:

1. Take a medium stockpot and place it over high heat.
2. Add butter and chicken broth to the pot and bring to a boil.
3. Break eggs into a bowl and beat them for 1 minute with a fork until frothy.
4. Once the broth boils, slowly pour in beaten eggs while stirring the broth with a spoon.
5. Cook for 1 minute with continuously stirring, then sprinkle salt and black pepper to season.
6. Garnish with sliced green onion, then serve warm.

Nutrition: Calories: 93 Fat: 7.8g Total carbs: 1.8g Fiber: 0.1g Protein: 3.9g

41. Cauliflower Cream Soup

Preparation Time: 15 minutes

Cooking Time: 4 hours 10 minutes

Servings: 5

Ingredients:

- 10 slices bacon
- 3 small heads cauliflower, cored and cut into florets
- 4 cups chicken broth
- ¼ cup (½ stick) salted butter
- 3 cloves garlic, pressed
- ½ large yellow onion, chopped
- 1 cup heavy whipping cream
- 2 cups Cheddar cheese, shredded
- Salt and black pepper, to taste
- Freshly chopped chives or green onions, for garnish

Directions:

1. Take a large skillet and place it over medium heat.
2. Add bacon to the skillet and cook for about 8 minutes until brown and crispy.
3. Transfer the cooked bacon to a paper towel-lined plate to absorb the excess grease.
4. Allow the bacon to cool, then chop it. Wrap the plate of chopped bacon in plastic and refrigerate it.
5. Add the cauliflower florets to the food processor and pulse until chopped thoroughly.
6. Add chicken broth, butter, garlic, onion, and chopped cauliflower to the slow cooker.

7. Give all these ingredients a gentle stir, then put on the lid.
8. Cook the cauliflower soup for 4 hours on high heat.
9. Once the cauliflower is tender, purée the soup with an immersion blender until smooth.
10. Add chopped bacon, heavy cream, cheese, salt, and black pepper. Mix well and let the cheese melt in the hot soup.
11. Garnish with green onions or chives, then serve warm.

Nutrition: Calories: 627 Fat: 54.3g Total carbs: 13.7g Fiber: 3.7g Protein: 24.6g

42. Shrimp Mushroom Chowder

Preparation Time: 10 minutes

Cooking Time: 40 minutes

Servings: 6

Ingredients:

- ¼ cup refined avocado oil
- 1/3 cup diced yellow onions
- 1 2/3 cups diced mushrooms
- 10½ ounces (298 g) small raw shrimp, shelled and deveined
- 1 can (131/2-ounce / 383-g) unsweetened coconut milk
- 1/3 cup chicken bone broth
- 2 tablespoons apple cider vinegar
- 1 teaspoon onion powder
- 1 teaspoon paprika
- 1 bay leaf
- ¾ teaspoon finely ground gray sea salt
- ½ teaspoon dried oregano leaves
- ¼ teaspoon ground black pepper
- 1 medium zucchini (7-ounce / 198-g), cubed
- 12 radishes (6-ounce / 170-g), cubed

Directions:

1. Add avocado oil to a large saucepan and place it over medium heat.
2. Add onions and mushrooms to the pan and sauté for 10 minutes or until onions are soft and mushrooms are lightly browned.

3. Stir in shrimp, coconut milk, chicken broth, apple cider vinegar, onion powder, paprika, bay leaf, sea salt, oregano leaves, and black pepper.
4. Cover the soup mixture with a lid and cook for 20 minutes on low heat.
5. Add zucchini and radishes to the soup and cook for 10 minutes.
6. Remove the bay leaf from the soup and divide the soup into 6 small serving bowls. Serve hot.

Nutrition: Calories: 311 Fat: 26.3g Total carbs: 7.7g Fiber: 2.9g Protein: 13.7g

43. Pork Tarragon Soup

Preparation Time: 10 minutes

Cooking Time: 1 hour 20 minutes

Servings: 6

Ingredients:

- 1/3 cup lard
- 1 pound (454 g) pork loin, cut into ½-inch (1.25-cm) pieces
- 10 strips bacon (about 10-ounce / 284-g), cut into ½-inch (1.25-cm) pieces
- ¾ cup sliced shallots
- 3 medium turnips (about 12½-ounce / 354-g), cubed
- 1 tablespoon yellow mustard
- ¼ cup dry white wine
- 1¾ cups chicken bone broth
- 4 sprigs fresh thyme
- 2 tablespoons unflavored gelatin
- 2 tablespoons apple cider vinegar
- ½ cup unsweetened coconut milk
- 1 tablespoon dried tarragon leaves

Directions:

1. Take a large saucepan and place it over medium heat.
2. Add lard to the saucepan and allow it to melt.
3. Add pork pieces to the melted lard and sauté for 8 minutes until golden brown.
4. Add bacon pieces and sliced shallots and sauté for 5 minutes or until fragrant.

5. Add turnips, mustard, wine, bone broth, and thyme sprigs to the soup.

6. Mix these ingredients gently and cover this soup with a lid.

7. Bring the soup to a boil, then reduce the heat to medium-low. Cook this soup for 1 hour.

8. Remove and discard the thyme sprigs from the soup then add gelatin, vinegar, coconut milk, and tarragon.

9. Increase the heat to medium and bring the soup to a boil. Cover to cook for 10 minutes.

10. Divide the cooked soup into 6 serving bowls and serve warm.

Nutrition: Calories: 566 Fat: 41.5g Total carbs: 9.7g Fiber: 1.2g Protein: 39.6g

SNACKS

44. Tempeh Tantrum Burgers

Preparation Time: 15 minutes

Cooking Time: 0 minutes

Servings: 4

Ingredients:

- 8 ounces tempeh, cut into 1⁄2-inch dice
- 3⁄4 cup chopped onion
- 2 garlic cloves, chopped
- 3⁄4 cup chopped walnuts
- 1⁄2 cup old-fashioned or quick-cooking oats
- tablespoon minced fresh parsley
- 1⁄2 teaspoon dried oregano
- 1⁄2 teaspoon dried thyme
- 1⁄2 teaspoon salt
- 1⁄4 teaspoon freshly ground black pepper
- tablespoons olive oil
- Dijon mustard
- whole-grain burger rolls
- Sliced red onion, tomato, lettuce, and avocado

Directions:

1. In a medium saucepan with simmering water, cook the tempeh for 30 minutes. Drain and set aside to cool.
2. In a food processor, combine together the onion and garlic and process until minced.

3. Put the cooled tempeh, the walnuts, oats, parsley, oregano, thyme, salt, and pepper. Process until well blended. Shape the mixture into 4 equal patties.
4. In a huge skillet, warm the oil at medium heat. Put the burgers and cook until cooked thoroughly and browned on both sides, about 7 minutes per side.
5. Spread the desired amount of mustard onto each half of the rolls and layer each roll with lettuce, tomato, red onion, and avocado, as desired. Serve immediately.

Nutrition: Calories: 372 kcal Protein: 16.3 g Fat: 28.49 g Carbohydrates: 17.4 g

45. Macadamia-Cashew Patties

Preparation Time: 10 minutes

Cooking Time: 10 minutes

Servings: 4

Ingredients:

- ¾ cup chopped macadamia nuts
- ¾ cup chopped cashews
- medium carrot, grated
- small onion, chopped
- garlic clove, minced
- jalapeño or other green Chile, seeded and minced
- ¾ cup old-fashioned oats
- ¾ cup dry unseasoned bread crumbs
- tablespoons minced fresh cilantro
- 1/2 teaspoon ground coriander
- Salt and freshly ground black pepper
- teaspoons fresh lime juice
- Canola or grapeseed oil, for frying
- sandwich rolls
- Lettuce leaves and condiment of choice

Directions:

1. In a food processor, combine together the macadamia nuts, cashews, carrot, onion, garlic, Chile, oats, bread crumbs, cilantro, coriander, and salt and pepper to taste. Process until well mixed. Add the lime juice and process until well blended. Taste, adjusting seasonings if necessary. Shape the mixture into 4 equal patties.

2. In a huge skillet, warm a thin layer of oil on medium heat. Put the patties and cook until golden brown on both sides, turning once about 10 minutes total. Serve on sandwich rolls with lettuce and condiments of choice.

Nutrition: Calories: 748 kcal Protein: 19.71 g Fat: 49.96 g Carbohydrates: 68.9 g

SMOOTHIES AND DRINKS

46. Strawberry Shake

Preparation Time: 5 minutes

Cooking Time: 0 minutes

Servings: 2

Ingredients:

- ½ cups almond milk
- ½ cup coconut milk, unsweetened or heavy whipping cream
- 5 ounces strawberries
- tablespoons sugar- free vanilla syrup
- tablespoons coconut oil
- Whipped cream or coconut cream, (optional)
- 2 tablespoons chia seeds (optional)

Directions:

1. Put all together the ingredients in a blender, and blend until you obtain a smooth mixture.
2. Put into tall glasses and serve topped with whipped cream if using.

Nutrition: Calories 276 Kcal Fat: 27.4 g Protein: 2.5 g Net carb: 6.4 g

47. Almond Smoothie

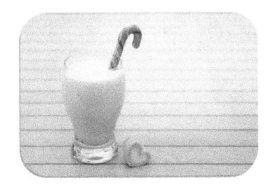

Preparation Time: 10 minutes

Cooking Time: 10 minutes

Servings: 2

Ingredients:

- ¾ cup almonds, chopped
- ½ cup heavy whipping cream
- 2 teaspoons butter, melted
- ¼ teaspoon organic vanilla extract
- 7–8 drops liquid stevia
- 1 cup unsweetened almond milk
- ¼ cup ice cubes

Directions:

1. In a blender, put all the listed **Ingredients:** and pulse until creamy.

2. Pour the smoothie into two glasses and serve immediately.

Nutrition: Calories 365 Net Carbs 4.5 g Total Fat 34.55 g Saturated Fat 10.8 g Cholesterol 51 mg Sodium 129 mg Total Carbs 9.5 g Fiber 5 g Sugar 1.6 g Protein 8.7 g

DRESSERTS

48. Vanilla Mug Cake

Preparation time: 5 minutes

Cooking time: 5 minutes

Servings: 1

Ingredients:

- tablespoon butter, melted
- tablespoons cream cheese
- tablespoons coconut flour
- tablespoon Swerve confectioners' style sweetener
- ½ teaspoon baking powder
- medium egg
- ¼ teaspoon liquid stevia
- drops vanilla extract
- 6 frozen raspberries

Directions:

1. Beat the butter with 2 tablespoons cream cheese in a mug, then place it in the microwave on high heat for about 1 minute until smooth.
2. Remove the mug from the microwave and let cool for 3 minutes.
3. Add the stevia, coconut flour, and baking powder, then mix again until the ingredients are well combined.
4. Add the Swerve, egg, and vanilla extract, and whisk while scraping down the sides of the mug. Put the

frozen raspberries on top and press them into the mixture.

5. Again, bake in the microwave on high heat for 1 minute and 20 seconds until the top springs back lightly when gently pressed with your fingertip.
6. Remove from the microwave and cool for 5 minutes before serving.

Nutrition: calories: 300 fat: 23.9g total carbs: 12.1g fiber: 0.8g protein: 9.9g

49. Chocolate Peanut Fudge

Preparation time: 10 minutes

Cooking time: 35 minutes

Servings: 12

Ingredients:

- 3½ ounces (99 g) dark chocolate with a minimum of 80% cocoa solids
- 4 tablespoons butter
- pinch salt
- ¼ cup peanut butter
- ½ teaspoon vanilla extract
- teaspoon ground cinnamon
- 1½ ounces (43 g) salted peanuts, finely chopped

Directions:

1. Mix the chocolate with butter in a microwave-safe bowl, and heat in the microwave oven or in a double boiler to melt.
2. When the chocolate is melted, stir well until it is smooth, and leave the mixture to cool.
3. Mix well and add the remaining ingredients except for nuts, then stir to combine.
4. Transfer this chocolate batter to a greased baking pan lined with parchment paper.
5. Top the batter with peanuts and chill in the refrigerator for 2 hours until firm.
6. Remove from the refrigerator and cut into squares to serve.

Nutrition: calories: 124 fat: 10.6g total carbs: 5.9g fiber: 1.6g protein: 2.9g

50. Carrot Cake

Preparation time: 10 minutes

Cooking time: 47 minutes

Servings: 6

Ingredients:

- Cooking oil spray, for greasing
- 3 eggs
- 4 ounces unsalted butter, melted
- 3 tablespoons low-carb sweetener, divided
- 2 teaspoons vanilla extract
- 2 cups grated or shredded carrots
- ⅓ cup chopped walnuts (optional)
- cup almond flour
- teaspoons pumpkin pie spice
- teaspoons baking powder
- 1½ cups water
- ounces cream cheese, room temperature

Directions:

1. Grease an 8-by-2-inch cake pan that fits in the pot with the cooking oil spray.
2. In a large bowl, use a hand mixer to beat the eggs, butter, 2 tablespoons of sweetener, and vanilla extract. Add the carrots and walnuts (if using) and stir to combine. Add the almond flour, pumpkin pie spice, and baking powder and stir until everything is combined. Pour the batter into the prepared cake pan.

3. Place the water in the pot. Place the reversible rack in the pot, making sure it is in the steam position. Place the pan on the rack. Assemble the pressure lid, making sure the pressure release valve is in the SEAL position.

4. When pressure cooking is complete, quick release the pressure by moving the pressure release valve to the VENT position. Carefully remove the lid when the unit has finished releasing pressure.

5. Carefully remove the cake from the pot. Let cool completely before frosting.

6. While the cake is cooling, place the cream cheese and remaining 1 tablespoon of sweetener in a medium bowl. Using a hand mixer, beat until the frosting is nice and fluffy. Once the cake has cooled, spread the frosting all over the top. Serve immediately or refrigerate until ready to serve.

Nutrition: Calories: 352; Total Fat: 32g; Total Carbohydrates: 8g; Fiber: 2g; Net Carbs: 6g; Protein: 8g; Erythritol Carbs: 6g Macronutrients: Fat: 82%; Protein: 9%; Carbs: 9%